Biomedical Innovation

Beyond the Horizon: Exploring the Transformative Frontier of Healthcare Advancements

Dr. Maya Thompson

Dedication

To all the brilliant minds dedicated to pushing the boundaries of biomedical innovation,

This book is dedicated to the tireless researchers, engineers, clinicians, and visionaries who strive to revolutionize healthcare. Your unwavering commitment, relentless pursuit of knowledge, and unwavering passion for improving lives inspire us all.

To the patients who bravely navigate their medical journeys, this dedication is for you. Your strength and resilience motivate us to never settle for the status quo and to continuously seek new breakthroughs that can bring hope and healing to those in need.

To my mentors and colleagues, thank you for your guidance, wisdom, and collaboration. Your insights and shared experiences have shaped my journey in biomedical innovation, and I am grateful for the opportunity to learn and grow alongside you.

Finally, to my family and loved ones, your unwavering support and belief in my dreams have been my foundation. This dedication is a testament to the love and encouragement that have fueled my pursuit of knowledge and the pursuit of a better future for all.

May this book serve as a beacon of inspiration, fostering creativity, collaboration, and the relentless pursuit of innovation in the field of biomedical science. Together, let us continue to push the boundaries and transform lives through the power of biomedical innovation.

With deep appreciation and boundless optimism,

Dr. Maya Thompson

Table of Contents

Introduction to Biomedical Innovation

Biomedical innovations, with their remarkable potential to transform healthcare, have emerged as a beacon of hope in the quest for improved patient outcomes and enhanced quality of life. These groundbreaking advancements at the intersection of biology, medicine, and technology are reshaping the landscape of healthcare delivery, paving the way for a future where diseases are better understood, treatments are more precise, and personalized therapies are the norm.

At its core, biomedical innovation encompasses a wide range of scientific and technological achievements that aim to tackle the complex challenges of human health. It brings together brilliant minds from diverse fields, including biology, genetics, engineering, computer science, and data analysis, fostering interdisciplinary collaborations that push the boundaries of knowledge and possibility.

The significance of biomedical innovations cannot be overstated. They hold the potential to revolutionize healthcare by offering new tools, approaches, and solutions to long standing medical problems. From cutting-edge technologies like gene editing, nanotechnology, and artificial intelligence to the advent of precision medicine, bioinformatics, and wearable devices, these innovations are catalysts for groundbreaking discoveries and transformative breakthroughs.

One of the most promising aspects of biomedical innovation lies in the realm of precision medicine. By leveraging advanced technologies like genomic sequencing, biomarker identification, and data analytics, precision medicine seeks to tailor treatments to individual patients based on their unique genetic makeup, lifestyle factors, and medical history. This personalized approach holds the promise of more effective treatments with fewer side effects, ultimately improving patient outcomes and quality of life.

Furthermore, the integration of bioinformatics and big data analytics has significantly accelerated the pace of biomedical research. The ability to analyze vast amounts of genetic and clinical data using machine learning algorithms has unlocked new insights into disease mechanisms, drug discovery, and clinical decision-making. This data-driven approach has the potential to revolutionize healthcare by enabling more accurate diagnoses, predictive modeling, and targeted therapies.

Biomedical innovation also encompasses the development of advanced medical devices and wearable technologies. These innovations enable remote patient monitoring, early disease detection, and personalized healthcare management. From smartwatches that track vital signs to implantable devices that deliver targeted therapies, these technologies empower patients to actively participate in their own healthcare and provide healthcare providers with real-time data for more informed decision-making.

Looking ahead, the field of biomedical innovation holds immense promise, but it also faces significant challenges. Translating research findings into clinical practice requires navigating complex regulatory frameworks, addressing ethical considerations, and ensuring accessibility and affordability of innovative treatments. Collaboration among scientists, clinicians, industry leaders, and policymakers is crucial to overcome these hurdles and ensure that biomedical innovations reach those who need them most.

In this book, we will delve into the fascinating world of biomedical innovation, exploring the latest breakthroughs, their impact on healthcare, and the future directions of this rapidly evolving field. Through the exploration of cutting-edge technologies, precision medicine, bioinformatics, bioprinting, and more, we aim to shed light on the transformative potential of biomedical innovation and inspire readers to embrace and engage with this exciting frontier of healthcare.

Together, we have the opportunity to reimagine healthcare delivery, empower patients, and revolutionize the way we prevent, diagnose, and treat diseases. Join us on this journey as we explore the awe-inspiring world of biomedical innovation and its profound significance in shaping the future of healthcare.

Biomedical innovations have the extraordinary potential to revolutionize healthcare, offering new avenues for improving patient outcomes and enhancing quality of life. These remarkable advancements, born at the intersection of biology, medicine, and technology, hold the promise of transforming the way we prevent, diagnose, and treat diseases, ultimately leading to a brighter and healthier future for individuals around the world.

At the heart of biomedical innovations lies the profound desire to improve the lives of patients. By pushing the boundaries of scientific knowledge and technological capabilities, researchers and innovators are paving the way for breakthroughs that have the power to change lives in remarkable ways. These innovations address the complex challenges of healthcare and aim to provide more effective, precise, and personalized treatments, thus improving patient outcomes and enhancing overall well-being.

One of the key areas where biomedical innovations have demonstrated their potential is in precision medicine. By unraveling the intricate tapestry of an individual's genetic makeup, lifestyle factors, and medical history, precision medicine brings forth an entirely new approach to healthcare. It allows for tailored treatments and interventions that are uniquely suited to each patient's specific needs, characteristics, and preferences. This personalized approach not only increases the likelihood of successful treatment outcomes but also minimizes the potential for adverse effects, ultimately improving patient well-being and quality of life.

Moreover, biomedical innovations in the field of diagnostics have the potential to revolutionize early disease detection and intervention. Advanced imaging technologies, high-throughput screening methods, and novel biomarker identification techniques enable the detection of diseases at their earliest stages, when interventions are most effective. By facilitating timely diagnosis, these innovations empower healthcare providers to initiate appropriate treatments promptly, leading to improved prognosis and better long-term outcomes for patients.

In addition to diagnostics and precision medicine, biomedical innovations are reshaping the landscape of treatment options. Novel therapeutic approaches, such as gene editing, targeted therapies, and regenerative medicine, are emerging as powerful tools in the fight against various diseases. By directly targeting disease-causing mechanisms, these innovations offer the potential for more effective and sustainable treatments, minimizing the burden of illness and enhancing the quality of life for patients.

Furthermore, the integration of technology into healthcare through biomedical innovations has opened up new possibilities for patient-centered care. Wearable devices, remote monitoring systems, and telemedicine platforms empower individuals to actively participate in their own healthcare management and provide healthcare providers with real-time data for more informed decision-making. This enhanced connectivity and patient engagement have the potential to improve treatment adherence, enable early intervention, and foster a collaborative approach between patients and healthcare professionals, ultimately leading to better health outcomes and improved quality of life.

As we embark on this journey through the realm of biomedical innovations, we will explore the cutting-edge technologies, breakthrough discoveries, and transformative approaches that hold the potential to revolutionize healthcare as we know it. By harnessing the power of biology, medicine, and technology, we can pave the way for a future where patients experience improved treatment outcomes, enhanced well-being, and a higher quality of life.

Join us as we delve into the captivating world of biomedical innovations and discover the endless possibilities they offer for transforming healthcare and making a positive impact on the lives of individuals worldwide. Together, let us embrace the potential of these innovations and work towards a future where better health and improved quality of life are within reach for all.

Foundations of Biomedical Innovation

Introduction:

Biomedical innovation has a rich and storied history, characterized by groundbreaking discoveries, transformative technologies, and the relentless pursuit of improving human health. In this chapter, we will embark on a journey through time to explore the historical development and key milestones that have shaped the field of biomedical innovation. Additionally, we will delve into the influential players and institutions that have been instrumental in driving biomedical research and development forward, pushing the boundaries of scientific knowledge and medical progress.

1.1 Historical Development:

Biomedical innovation can trace its roots back to ancient civilizations, where early medical practices and knowledge laid the foundation for future advancements. From the ancient Egyptians' pioneering efforts in surgery to the Ayurvedic medicine of ancient India and the Greek physician Hippocrates' contributions to medical ethics, these early developments paved the way for the emergence of modern biomedical innovation.

The Renaissance period witnessed a remarkable resurgence in scientific inquiry and medical advancements. Figures such as Leonardo da Vinci, with his anatomical drawings, and Andreas Vesalius, who revolutionized the study of human anatomy, made significant contributions to the understanding of the human body. This period marked a turning point, as empirical observation and evidence-based medicine became increasingly influential.

The 19th and 20th centuries witnessed unprecedented progress in biomedical innovation. The discovery of the germ theory of disease by Louis Pasteur and Robert Koch revolutionized our understanding of infectious diseases and led to significant developments in sanitation, vaccination, and antimicrobial therapies. The advent of anesthesia and antiseptics spurred advancements in surgical techniques, enabling more complex procedures and reducing patient suffering.

The mid-20th century brought about a new era of biomedical innovation, with the discovery of DNA structure by James Watson and Francis Crick and the subsequent unraveling of the genetic code. This breakthrough laid the foundation for modern genetics, molecular biology, and the field of genomics, which have had a transformative impact on medicine, leading to personalized treatments and precision medicine approaches.

1.2 Key Players and Institutions:

Biomedical research and development are driven by a diverse array of visionary individuals and institutions. In the academic realm, universities and research institutes play a pivotal role in fostering scientific discovery and innovation. Institutions such as Harvard Medical School, the National Institutes of Health (NIH), and the Max Planck Society have been at the forefront of biomedical research, producing groundbreaking discoveries and nurturing generations of scientists.

Pharmaceutical and biotechnology companies are key players in advancing biomedical innovation. Companies like Pfizer, Johnson & Johnson, Novartis, and Amgen invest heavily in research and development, driving the translation of scientific discoveries into tangible therapies and medical interventions. These industry players bring together multidisciplinary teams of scientists, engineers, and clinicians to develop innovative drugs, medical devices, and therapies that address unmet medical needs.

Government agencies and regulatory bodies also play a crucial role in shaping the landscape of biomedical innovation. The U.S. Food and Drug Administration (FDA), the European Medicines Agency (EMA), and similar organizations worldwide ensure the safety and efficacy of medical products, while also fostering an environment conducive to innovation and scientific progress.

In addition to these key players, philanthropic organizations, such as the Bill and Melinda Gates Foundation and the Wellcome Trust, contribute significantly to biomedical innovation. Through their funding and support, they drive research initiatives, promote global health, and address pressing healthcare challenges.

Conclusion:
The historical development of biomedical innovation is a testament to human curiosity, ingenuity, and the relentless pursuit of improving healthcare outcomes. From ancient civilizations to the modern era, visionary individuals, academic institutions, industry leaders, and government agencies have all played critical roles in advancing biomedical research and development.

As we move forward, this historical groundwork serves as a launching pad for future breakthroughs. The collaborative efforts of these key players and institutions, combined with advances in technology and scientific knowledge, continue to shape the field of biomedical innovation, propelling us toward a future where diseases are better understood, treatments are more effective, and the health and well-being of individuals are significantly improved.

Key Players and Institutions Driving Biomedical Research and Development

Biomedical research and development are driven by a diverse range of key players and institutions that contribute significantly to advancing scientific knowledge, discovering breakthroughs, and translating innovative ideas into tangible medical solutions. These players and institutions collaborate, innovate, and invest in biomedical research to push the boundaries of healthcare and improve patient outcomes. Let's explore some of the prominent actors in the field.

1. Academic Institutions:

Academic institutions, including universities and research centers, play a pivotal role in driving biomedical research. These institutions foster an environment of intellectual curiosity and scientific inquiry, providing a platform for researchers and scientists to explore novel ideas and pursue groundbreaking discoveries. Institutions such as Harvard Medical School, Stanford University School of Medicine, Johns Hopkins University School of Medicine, and the University of Oxford have a long-standing reputation for their contributions to biomedical research and their ability to attract top talent.

2. Government Agencies and Funding Bodies:
Government agencies and funding bodies significantly contribute to biomedical research and development by providing financial support, infrastructure, and regulatory frameworks. The National Institutes of Health (NIH) in the United States, the European Commission, the Medical Research Council (MRC) in the United Kingdom, and similar organizations worldwide fund research projects, support scientific collaborations, and promote innovation in healthcare. These agencies also establish guidelines and regulations to ensure the safety and ethical conduct of biomedical research.

3. Pharmaceutical and Biotechnology Companies:
Pharmaceutical and biotechnology companies are major players in driving biomedical research and development. These companies invest heavily in research, employing scientists, clinicians, and engineers to explore new therapeutic approaches, develop innovative drugs, and design cutting-edge medical devices. Industry leaders such as Pfizer, Johnson & Johnson, Novartis, Roche, and Amgen have the resources, expertise, and infrastructure to conduct clinical trials, navigate regulatory processes, and bring life-saving therapies to market. Their contributions are instrumental in translating scientific discoveries into tangible medical solutions that benefit patients worldwide.

4. Philanthropic Organizations:

Philanthropic organizations play a vital role in driving biomedical research by providing substantial financial support, resources, and expertise. Organizations like the Bill and Melinda Gates Foundation, the Wellcome Trust, the Howard Hughes Medical Institute, and the Chan Zuckerberg Initiative invest in initiatives that address global health challenges, support innovative research projects, and foster collaborations between academia, industry, and healthcare providers. Their philanthropic efforts have a transformative impact on biomedical research and help address health disparities worldwide.

5. Collaborative Research Networks:

Collaborative research networks bring together scientists, clinicians, and industry partners from various institutions and disciplines to work collectively on biomedical research projects. These networks facilitate knowledge sharing, enhance research capabilities, and promote interdisciplinary collaborations. Examples of collaborative research networks include the International Cancer Genome Consortium (ICGC), the Global Alliance for Genomics and Health (GA4GH), and the Human Cell Atlas (HCA) project. These networks leverage collective expertise and resources to accelerate discoveries and drive advancements in healthcare.

Conclusion:

The landscape of biomedical research and development is shaped by a diverse array of key players and institutions. Academic institutions foster scientific curiosity and provide the infrastructure for research. Government agencies and funding bodies offer financial support and establish regulatory frameworks. Pharmaceutical and biotechnology companies drive innovation and bring therapies to market. Philanthropic organizations provide resources and support initiatives addressing global health challenges. Collaborative research networks facilitate interdisciplinary collaborations. Together, these key players and institutions drive biomedical research and development, pushing the boundaries of knowledge and technology to improve healthcare outcomes and enhance the well-being of individuals worldwide.

Ethical Considerations and Regulatory Frameworks Surrounding Biomedical Innovation

Biomedical innovation brings forth remarkable advancements in healthcare, with the potential to improve patient outcomes and enhance quality of life. However, the development and implementation of these innovations also raise important ethical considerations that must be carefully addressed. In addition, regulatory frameworks play a crucial role in ensuring the safety, efficacy, and ethical conduct of biomedical research and the translation of innovative ideas into clinical practice. Let's explore some of the key ethical considerations and regulatory frameworks in the field of biomedical innovation.

1. Informed Consent and Patient Autonomy:
Respecting individual autonomy and obtaining informed consent are fundamental ethical principles in biomedical research and innovation. Informed consent ensures that individuals are fully informed about the nature, risks, and potential benefits of their participation in research or treatment. It allows individuals to make autonomous decisions based on their values, preferences, and understanding of the potential outcomes. Ethical guidelines and regulatory frameworks require researchers and healthcare

providers to obtain informed consent from participants and patients before involving them in research studies or providing innovative treatments.

2. Privacy and Data Protection:

The collection, storage, and use of personal health information and genomic data raise important ethical and legal considerations. Biomedical innovation often relies on the analysis of sensitive and personal data, which must be handled with utmost care to protect individuals' privacy. Regulatory frameworks, such as the General Data Protection Regulation (GDPR) in the European Union, establish guidelines for the lawful and ethical handling of personal data, ensuring that data is collected and used in a transparent and secure manner. Researchers and healthcare institutions must adhere to strict data protection protocols to safeguard patient privacy and maintain confidentiality.

3. Ethical Use of Human Subjects:

Biomedical research involving human subjects must adhere to ethical principles to protect their welfare and ensure the validity of research outcomes. Institutional review boards (IRBs) or ethics committees play a crucial role in evaluating research protocols, assessing potential risks and benefits, and ensuring that studies comply with ethical guidelines. These bodies review research proposals, monitor ongoing studies, and make decisions regarding the ethical appropriateness of research involving human subjects. Ethical considerations include minimizing harm, maximizing benefits, ensuring equitable distribution of benefits and burdens, and addressing potential conflicts of interest.

4. Responsible Innovation and Risk Assessment:

Biomedical innovation must be accompanied by a thorough assessment of potential risks, both to individual patients and to society as a whole. Regulatory frameworks require researchers and innovators to conduct rigorous risk assessments before introducing new technologies or treatments. This includes evaluating the safety and efficacy of interventions, considering potential long-term effects, and weighing the benefits against the risks. Ethical considerations also encompass responsible innovation, which involves anticipating and addressing the potential social, economic, and ethical implications of new technologies, such as their impact on healthcare disparities, access to care, and the potential for unintended consequences.

5. Regulatory Oversight and Compliance:

Regulatory frameworks, such as those enforced by the U.S. Food and Drug Administration (FDA), the European Medicines Agency (EMA), and similar bodies worldwide, play a crucial role in ensuring the safety, efficacy, and ethical conduct of biomedical research and the development of innovative therapies.

These regulatory bodies review and approve clinical trials, evaluate the safety and effectiveness of new drugs and medical devices, and monitor the post-marketing surveillance of products in use. Compliance with regulatory requirements is essential to protect patient safety, maintain public trust, and ensure that biomedical innovations meet the highest ethical standards.

Conclusion:
Ethical considerations and regulatory frameworks are integral to the responsible development and implementation of biomedical innovations. By addressing these considerations and adhering to regulatory guidelines, researchers, healthcare providers, and innovators can navigate the complex landscape of biomedical innovation while upholding fundamental ethical principles, protecting patient rights, and ensuring the safety and well-being of individuals. Balancing scientific progress with ethical considerations and robust regulatory oversight is essential to foster trust, promote patient-centered care, and maximize the potential benefits of biomedical innovation for society as a whole.

Cutting-Edge Technologies in Biomedical Innovation

Biomedical innovation is continuously propelled forward by cutting-edge technologies that revolutionize the way we understand, diagnose, and treat diseases. In recent years, several remarkable advancements have emerged, transforming the field of healthcare. In this chapter, we will explore three groundbreaking technologies: gene editing, nanotechnology, and artificial intelligence (AI), and their impact on biomedical innovation.

1. Gene Editing:

Gene editing is a powerful technology that allows scientists to precisely modify the DNA of living organisms. One of the most notable gene editing techniques is CRISPR-Cas9, which has revolutionized the field with its simplicity and versatility. CRISPR-Cas9 enables researchers to edit genes by precisely targeting specific DNA sequences and introducing desired changes. This technology has the potential to correct genetic mutations associated with inherited diseases, enhance the understanding of disease mechanisms, and develop new therapies.

Gene editing also holds promise for personalized medicine, as it allows for the customization of treatments to an individual's genetic makeup. By targeting specific genes or gene pathways, scientists can develop therapies that are tailored to a patient's unique genetic profile, potentially improving treatment outcomes and minimizing adverse effects. However, ethical considerations surrounding gene editing, particularly in germline editing, continue to be a topic of debate and require careful consideration.

2. Nanotechnology:
Nanotechnology involves the manipulation and control of matter at the nanoscale, typically at dimensions of 1 to 100 nanometers. In biomedicine, nanotechnology offers exciting possibilities for targeted drug delivery, diagnostics, and regenerative medicine. Nanoparticles can be engineered to carry drugs or therapeutic agents, allowing for precise and controlled release at specific sites in the body. This targeted drug delivery approach improves drug efficacy while minimizing systemic side effects.

Nanotechnology also plays a crucial role in diagnostic techniques, enabling highly sensitive and specific detection of diseases. Nanosensors and nanomaterials can be designed to detect biomarkers or abnormal cellular activities, facilitating early disease detection and monitoring. Additionally, nanotechnology-based tissue engineering approaches hold promise for regenerative medicine, where engineered nanomaterials can provide structural support and promote tissue regeneration.

3. Artificial Intelligence (AI):

Artificial intelligence has become a transformative technology in biomedical innovation. AI algorithms can process vast amounts of data, identify patterns, and generate insights that aid in diagnosis, treatment planning, and drug discovery. Machine learning, a subset of AI, allows computers to learn from data and improve their performance over time.

In healthcare, AI-powered systems can analyze medical images, such as X-rays, MRIs, and CT scans, to assist radiologists in detecting abnormalities and making accurate diagnoses. AI algorithms can also predict disease outcomes, assess the risk of complications, and aid in personalized treatment decisions based on individual patient characteristics. Additionally, AI algorithms are being used to analyze large-scale genomics and proteomics datasets, helping to unravel the complexities of diseases and identify potential drug targets.

However, ethical considerations surrounding AI in healthcare include data privacy, transparency, and the potential for algorithmic bias. Ensuring the responsible development and deployment of AI technologies in healthcare is crucial to maintain trust, protect patient privacy, and mitigate unintended consequences.

Conclusion:
Gene editing, nanotechnology, and artificial intelligence are revolutionizing biomedical innovation, offering unprecedented opportunities to understand, diagnose, and treat diseases. These cutting-edge technologies hold the potential to transform healthcare by enabling precise genetic modifications, targeted drug delivery, early disease detection, and personalized treatment approaches. However, their ethical implications, regulatory considerations, and responsible implementation must be carefully addressed to harness their full potential and ensure their safe and ethical integration into clinical practice. With continued advancements and interdisciplinary collaborations, these technologies will continue to shape the future of biomedical innovation, paving the way for improved patient outcomes and a deeper understanding of human health and disease.

Cutting-Edge Technologies in Biomedical Innovation

Cutting-edge technologies in biomedical innovation, such as gene editing, nanotechnology, and artificial intelligence (AI), have the potential to revolutionize disease diagnosis, treatment, and prevention. These technologies offer exciting possibilities for improving healthcare outcomes, enhancing personalized medicine approaches, and advancing our understanding of diseases. In this chapter, we will explore their potential applications in these critical areas.

1. Disease Diagnosis:

a. Gene Editing: Gene editing technologies, like CRISPR-Cas9, can aid in disease diagnosis by enabling precise and efficient detection of genetic mutations associated with various disorders. CRISPR-based diagnostic platforms can be designed to recognize specific genetic sequences or variations, providing rapid and accurate identification of disease-related genetic markers. These tools hold promise for early detection and screening of genetic diseases.

b. Nanotechnology: Nanotechnology-based diagnostic approaches offer sensitive and specific detection of disease biomarkers, facilitating early diagnosis and monitoring. Nanosensors and nanomaterials can be engineered to recognize and bind to specific molecules or abnormal cellular activities associated with diseases. This enables the development of highly sensitive diagnostic tests that detect diseases at an early stage, allowing for timely interventions and improved patient outcomes.

c. Artificial Intelligence: AI algorithms can analyze large datasets, including medical images and patient records, to aid in disease diagnosis. AI-powered image analysis systems can assist radiologists in detecting abnormalities in medical images, improving the accuracy and efficiency of diagnosis. AI algorithms can also integrate multiple data sources and identify patterns that may be indicative of specific diseases, contributing to more precise and timely diagnoses.

2. Disease Treatment:
a. Gene Editing: Gene editing technologies hold promise for developing novel therapies by correcting disease-causing genetic mutations. By precisely modifying the DNA, gene editing can potentially address the root cause of genetic disorders. This approach has the potential to revolutionize the treatment of inherited diseases, offering hope for conditions that were previously untreatable or had limited treatment options.

b. Nanotechnology: Nanotechnology enables targeted drug delivery, enhancing the efficacy and safety of treatments. Nanoparticles can be designed to carry drugs or therapeutic agents to specific sites in the body, allowing for precise delivery and minimizing systemic side effects. This targeted approach improves treatment outcomes and reduces the toxicity associated with conventional therapies.

c. Artificial Intelligence: AI can assist in treatment planning and personalized medicine approaches. AI algorithms can analyze patient data, including genetic information, medical history, and treatment outcomes, to identify the most effective treatment options for individual patients. This enables healthcare providers to make data-driven decisions, optimizing treatment strategies and improving patient outcomes.

3. Disease Prevention:
a. Gene Editing: Gene editing technologies have the potential to prevent the transmission of genetic diseases to future generations. By editing disease-causing genetic mutations in reproductive cells or embryos, gene editing can eliminate the risk of passing on inherited disorders to offspring. However, ethical considerations surrounding germline gene editing and its long-term implications require careful evaluation and societal discussion.

b.   Nanotechnology: Nanotechnology   offers opportunities for targeted drug delivery of preventive interventions. By delivering vaccines or prophylactic agents directly to specific cells or tissues, nanotechnology can enhance the immune response and improve the effectiveness of preventive measures. This approach holds promise for preventing infectious diseases and reducing the burden of epidemics.

c. Artificial Intelligence: AI can contribute to disease prevention through predictive analytics and risk assessment. By analyzing large-scale datasets and identifying patterns, AI algorithms can predict disease risk and stratify individuals based on their susceptibility to certain conditions. This information can inform preventive interventions, lifestyle modifications, and personalized screening programs, leading to early detection and intervention.

Conclusion:
Gene editing, nanotechnology, and artificial intelligence have immense potential in disease diagnosis, treatment, and prevention. These cutting-edge technologies offer innovative approaches to identify diseases at an early stage, develop targeted therapies, and personalize treatment strategies. By harnessing the power of these technologies, we can improve healthcare outcomes, enhance disease prevention efforts, and pave the way for a future of

more precise and effective healthcare interventions. However, the ethical considerations, regulatory frameworks, and responsible implementation of these technologies must be carefully addressed to ensure their safe and ethical integration into clinical practice and maximize their potential benefits for individuals and society.

Cutting-Edge Technologies in Biomedical Innovation

One of the most remarkable aspects of cutting-edge technologies in biomedical innovation, including gene editing, nanotechnology, and artificial intelligence (AI), is their transformative impact on healthcare. These technologies have brought about numerous success stories and case studies that highlight their potential to revolutionize disease management, improve patient outcomes, and advance medical research. In this chapter, we will explore some of these notable examples.

1. Gene Editing:

a. Case Study: Sickle Cell Disease Treatment - In 2019, a groundbreaking case highlighted the potential of gene editing in treating genetic disorders. A patient with sickle cell disease received an experimental gene therapy using CRISPR-Cas9 to edit the patient's own stem cells. The therapy aimed to correct the underlying genetic mutation responsible for the disease. The patient's edited cells were then reintroduced into their body, leading to a significant reduction in the symptoms of sickle cell disease. This case demonstrated the potential of gene editing as a curative approach for genetic diseases.

b. Success Story: HIV Resistance - Another success story in gene editing involves HIV resistance. Researchers used CRISPR-Cas9 to modify the CCR5 gene in human immune cells, rendering them resistant to HIV infection. This gene editing approach opens up the possibility of providing long-term protection against HIV and has the potential to revolutionize the prevention and treatment of this devastating disease.

2. Nanotechnology:

a. Case Study: Targeted Drug Delivery - Nanotechnology has revolutionized drug delivery by enabling targeted and controlled release of therapeutic agents. One notable case involved the use of nanotechnology to treat cancer. Scientists developed nanoparticles that could carry chemotherapy drugs directly to tumor sites while sparing healthy tissues. This targeted drug delivery approach enhanced the efficacy of the treatment and reduced the systemic side effects traditionally associated with chemotherapy.

b. Success Story: Point-of-Care Diagnostics - Nanotechnology-based point-of-care diagnostics have become instrumental in improving disease diagnosis, especially in resource-limited settings. For instance, a portable nanotechnology-based diagnostic device was developed to detect malaria infections quickly and accurately. The device utilizes nanosensors to detect malaria-specific biomarkers in blood samples, providing rapid results that aid in timely treatment and control of the disease.

3. Artificial Intelligence:

a. Case Study: AI in Radiology - AI algorithms have made significant strides in radiology, assisting radiologists in the interpretation of medical images. In a case study, an AI algorithm was trained to analyze mammograms for breast cancer detection. The algorithm achieved a level of accuracy comparable to that of expert radiologists, demonstrating the potential of AI in improving diagnostic accuracy and efficiency.

b. Success Story: Predictive Analytics for Patient Outcomes - AI has proven to be a valuable tool in predicting patient outcomes and guiding treatment decisions. For example, researchers developed an AI-based predictive model that analyzed patient data and predicted the likelihood of sepsis, a life-threatening infection. The model allowed healthcare providers to identify at-risk patients earlier, initiate appropriate interventions, and improve patient outcomes.

These case studies and success stories illustrate the transformative power of gene editing, nanotechnology, and artificial intelligence in healthcare. They demonstrate how these technologies have the potential to revolutionize disease treatment, enhance diagnostic accuracy, and improve patient care. While further research and development are still needed, these advancements serve as promising indicators of what the future holds for biomedical innovation and its impact on healthcare.

Precision Medicine and Personalized Therapies

The emergence of precision medicine has ushered in a new era of healthcare delivery, transforming the way diseases are diagnosed, treated, and managed. Precision medicine aims to tailor medical interventions to individual patients based on their unique genetic, environmental, and lifestyle factors. By taking into account the specific characteristics of each patient, precision medicine enables more targeted and effective therapies, leading to improved patient outcomes. In this chapter, we will discuss the emergence of precision medicine and its impact on healthcare delivery.

1. Advancements in Genomics:

One of the key drivers behind precision medicine is the rapid progress in genomics research. The Human Genome Project and subsequent advancements in DNA sequencing technologies have made it possible to analyze an individual's genetic blueprint with unprecedented accuracy and speed. This has led to a deeper understanding of the genetic basis of diseases and the identification of genetic variants associated with various conditions.

2. Personalized Diagnostics:

Precision medicine has revolutionized disease diagnostics by enabling the identification of specific biomarkers and genetic mutations associated with diseases. By analyzing a patient's genetic profile or molecular signatures, healthcare providers can make more accurate and timely diagnoses. This allows for early detection of diseases and the implementation of personalized treatment strategies.

3. Targeted Therapies:

Precision medicine has led to the development of targeted therapies that focus on the specific molecular or genetic alterations driving a patient's disease. These therapies are designed to selectively target and inhibit the molecules or pathways involved in the disease process, while sparing healthy tissues. Targeted therapies have shown remarkable success in treating cancers, autoimmune disorders, and rare genetic diseases, among others.

4. Pharmacogenomics:

Pharmacogenomics, a branch of precision medicine, examines how an individual's genetic makeup affects their response to medications. By analyzing genetic variants that influence drug metabolism and efficacy, healthcare providers can optimize medication selection and dosage for each patient. This approach minimizes adverse drug reactions, improves treatment outcomes, and reduces the trial-and-error process often associated with medication selection.

5. Prevention and Risk Assessment:

Precision medicine emphasizes proactive approaches to disease prevention and risk assessment. By analyzing an individual's genetic predisposition, lifestyle factors, and environmental exposures, healthcare providers can assess an individual's risk for developing certain diseases. This information can guide personalized prevention strategies, such as lifestyle modifications, targeted screening programs, and early interventions to mitigate disease risk.

6. Data Integration and Artificial Intelligence:

Precision medicine heavily relies on the integration of vast amounts of patient data, including genetic information, electronic health records, and clinical outcomes. Artificial intelligence (AI) algorithms play a crucial role in analyzing and interpreting these complex datasets. AI can identify patterns, predict disease outcomes, and assist healthcare providers in making more informed decisions regarding treatment plans and patient management.

7. Ethical Considerations and Challenges:

While precision medicine holds tremendous promise, it also presents ethical considerations and challenges.

Issues such as data privacy, informed consent, equitable access to therapies, and the responsible use of genetic information require careful attention. Robust ethical frameworks and policies must be established to ensure the responsible implementation of precision medicine and to address potential ethical concerns.

In conclusion, precision medicine has emerged as a transformative approach to healthcare delivery. By leveraging advances in genomics, personalized diagnostics, targeted therapies, pharmacogenomics, and data integration, precision medicine enables tailored interventions that consider the unique characteristics of each patient. This approach holds great potential for improving patient outcomes, enhancing disease prevention efforts, and optimizing healthcare delivery. However, ethical considerations, regulatory frameworks, and the responsible use of patient data are crucial in realizing the full potential of precision medicine while ensuring equitable and ethical healthcare practices.

Precision Medicine and Personalized Therapies

The field of precision medicine has witnessed significant advancements in recent years, driven by the integration of genomic sequencing, biomarker identification, and data analytics. These powerful tools have revolutionized healthcare by enabling the development of personalized therapies tailored to the individual characteristics of patients. In this chapter, we will explore how genomic sequencing, biomarker identification, and data analytics contribute to the realization of personalized therapies.

1. Genomic Sequencing:

Genomic sequencing, the process of determining the complete DNA sequence of an individual, lies at the core of precision medicine. Technological advancements have made it possible to rapidly and cost-effectively sequence an individual's entire genome or specific regions of interest. Genomic sequencing provides a comprehensive view of an individual's genetic makeup, uncovering variations and mutations that may contribute to disease susceptibility or treatment response.

2. Biomarker Identification:

Biomarkers play a crucial role in guiding personalized therapies. These are measurable indicators, such as genetic variations, proteins, or other molecules, that can be used to assess disease status, predict treatment response, or monitor therapeutic efficacy. Genomic sequencing and other molecular profiling techniques enable the identification of biomarkers associated with specific diseases or treatment outcomes. Biomarkers serve as valuable tools for tailoring therapies to individual patients, ensuring more precise and effective treatments.

3. Data Analytics:

The vast amount of data generated from genomic sequencing, biomarker identification, and patient records necessitates sophisticated data analytics tools to extract meaningful insights. Data analytics techniques, including machine learning and artificial intelligence, are employed to analyze complex datasets, identify patterns, and make predictions. These tools enable healthcare providers to integrate and interpret diverse sources of information, leading to more informed decision-making regarding treatment selection, dosage optimization, and patient management.

4. Personalized Therapies:

The integration of genomic sequencing, biomarker identification, and data analytics facilitates the development of personalized therapies. Here are some examples of how these technologies enable personalized treatments:

a. Targeted Therapies: Genomic sequencing and biomarker identification help identify specific mutations or molecular alterations driving a patient's disease. This information allows for the development of targeted therapies that selectively inhibit the disease-causing molecules or pathways. Targeted therapies have shown remarkable success in treating various cancers, where specific genomic alterations guide the selection of appropriate drugs.

b. Pharmacogenomics: Genomic sequencing can reveal genetic variations that affect an individual's response to medications. Pharmacogenomics, the study of how genetic factors influence drug response, enables personalized medication selection and dosage adjustment. By considering an individual's genetic profile, healthcare providers can optimize treatment outcomes while minimizing the risk of adverse drug reactions.

c. Immunotherapies: Biomarker identification plays a crucial role in the field of immunotherapy. Biomarkers, such as specific gene expression patterns or immune cell profiles, help predict which patients are most likely to respond to immunotherapies. This enables the selection of patients who are more likely to benefit from these treatments, optimizing therapeutic efficacy.

d. Disease Monitoring: Biomarkers identified through genomic sequencing and other molecular profiling techniques can be used to monitor disease progression and treatment response. Regular monitoring of biomarkers allows healthcare providers to adjust treatment plans in real-time, ensuring that therapies remain targeted and effective.

5. Advancing Research and Clinical Trials:
The integration of genomic sequencing, biomarker identification, and data analytics also enhances research and clinical trials. By stratifying patients based on their genetic profiles and biomarker status, researchers can conduct more focused and efficient clinical trials. This approach increases the likelihood of identifying patient subgroups that respond favorably to specific therapies, accelerating the development of novel treatments and improving patient outcomes.

In conclusion, the integration of genomic sequencing, biomarker identification, and data analytics has paved the way for personalized therapies in precision medicine. These technologies enable the precise characterization of diseases, identification of relevant biomarkers, and the development of tailored treatments. By leveraging the power of genomics and data analytics, healthcare providers can offer patients more effective and targeted therapies, leading to improved treatment outcomes and a shift towards personalized healthcare.

Precision Medicine and Personalized Therapies

Implementing personalized medicine approaches, such as precision medicine, holds great promise for revolutionizing healthcare. By tailoring medical interventions to individual patients based on their unique characteristics, personalized medicine aims to improve treatment outcomes, enhance disease prevention, and optimize healthcare delivery. However, along with its numerous benefits, there are also challenges that need to be addressed. In this chapter, we will highlight the benefits and challenges in implementing personalized medicine approaches.

Benefits of Personalized Medicine:

1. Targeted and Effective Treatments: Personalized medicine allows for the development of targeted therapies that address the specific molecular and genetic alterations driving a patient's disease. By tailoring treatments to individual characteristics, healthcare providers can maximize therapeutic efficacy while minimizing adverse effects.

2. Precision Diagnostics: Personalized medicine emphasizes the use of advanced diagnostic techniques, such as genomic sequencing and biomarker

identification, to accurately diagnose diseases and predict treatment responses. This enables early detection of diseases and the implementation of timely and targeted interventions.

3. Improved Patient Outcomes: By considering individual patient characteristics, personalized medicine has the potential to significantly improve patient outcomes. Tailored treatments increase the likelihood of positive responses and reduce the risk of treatment failures, leading to better clinical outcomes and enhanced quality of life for patients.

4. Disease Prevention and Risk Assessment: Personalized medicine emphasizes proactive approaches to disease prevention. By integrating genetic, environmental, and lifestyle factors, healthcare providers can assess an individual's disease risk and develop personalized prevention strategies. This approach has the potential to reduce disease incidence and improve population health.

5. Advancements in Research and Drug Development: Personalized medicine approaches generate vast amounts of data, including genomic and clinical information, which can be leveraged to advance medical research and drug development. By stratifying patients based on their unique characteristics, researchers can conduct more targeted clinical trials,

leading to the identification of patient subgroups that respond favorably to specific treatments.

Challenges in Implementing Personalized Medicine:

1. Complex Data Integration: Personalized medicine relies on the integration of diverse data sources, including genomic sequencing data, electronic health records, and biomarker information. The challenge lies in effectively managing and integrating these complex datasets to derive meaningful insights and guide clinical decision-making.

2. Cost and Accessibility: The implementation of personalized medicine approaches can be costly, particularly in terms of genomic sequencing and advanced diagnostic techniques. The cost-effectiveness and accessibility of these technologies need to be addressed to ensure equitable access to personalized therapies for all patients.

3. Ethical and Privacy Concerns: Personalized medicine involves the collection and analysis of sensitive patient data, raising ethical and privacy concerns. Strict guidelines and regulations must be in place to protect patient privacy, ensure informed consent, and prevent any misuse or unauthorized access to sensitive genetic and health information.

4. Integration into Clinical Practice: Integrating personalized medicine approaches into routine clinical practice can pose challenges. Healthcare providers need to be trained in interpreting and utilizing genomic and biomarker information effectively. Additionally, healthcare systems must be equipped with the necessary infrastructure and resources to implement personalized medicine approaches.

5. Limited Evidence and Validation: Personalized medicine is still a relatively young field, and the evidence base supporting its implementation for various diseases and conditions is evolving. Further research and validation are needed to establish the efficacy, safety, and cost-effectiveness of personalized medicine approaches across different patient populations and healthcare settings.

In conclusion, implementing personalized medicine approaches offers significant benefits in terms of targeted treatments, precise diagnostics, improved patient outcomes, disease prevention, and advancements in research. However, challenges related to data integration, cost and accessibility, ethical considerations, integration into clinical practice, and limited evidence need to be addressed. Overcoming these challenges will require collaborative efforts from healthcare providers, researchers, policymakers, and industry stakeholders. By addressing these challenges, personalized medicine has the potential to transform healthcare, leading to more effective and patient-centered approaches to disease management and prevention.

Bioinformatics and Big Data Analytics in Biomedical Research

Bioinformatics and big data analytics have emerged as critical components in advancing biomedical research. In this chapter, we will explore the pivotal role of bioinformatics and big data analytics in accelerating discoveries, fostering innovation, and transforming healthcare.

1. Data Integration and Management:
Bioinformatics and big data analytics provide the means to integrate and manage vast and diverse datasets generated in biomedical research. These datasets encompass genomic sequences, clinical records, imaging data, and more. By harmonizing and linking different types of data, researchers can gain a comprehensive understanding of diseases, identify new biomarkers, and uncover potential therapeutic targets.

2. Genomic Analysis and Variant Interpretation:
Bioinformatics plays a crucial role in analyzing genomic data, particularly DNA sequencing data. With the aid of advanced algorithms, researchers can identify genetic variations associated with diseases,

assess their functional impact, and interpret their clinical relevance. This enables the identification of disease-causing mutations, the discovery of genetic predispositions, and the development of personalized treatment strategies.

3. Transcriptomics and Proteomics:

Bioinformatics tools facilitate the analysis of transcriptomic and proteomic data, providing insights into gene expression patterns and protein interactions. Through sophisticated algorithms, researchers can identify disease-specific biomarkers, elucidate molecular pathways, and uncover potential drug targets. This knowledge contributes to the development of targeted therapies and precision medicine approaches.

4. Data Mining and Knowledge Discovery:

Big data analytics in bioinformatics involves data mining and knowledge discovery from large-scale datasets. Machine learning algorithms can identify patterns, correlations, and hidden relationships within complex biological systems. By analyzing diverse data sources such as genomic data, electronic health records, and scientific literature, researchers can uncover novel associations, identify predictive models, and gain deeper insights into disease mechanisms.

5. Predictive Modeling and Clinical Decision Support:

Bioinformatics, in conjunction with machine learning algorithms, enables the development of predictive models and clinical decision support systems. By utilizing large-scale data, including clinical records, genetic profiles, and treatment outcomes, researchers can create models that predict disease progression, treatment responses, and patient outcomes. These models aid healthcare providers in making informed decisions, tailoring treatment strategies, and improving patient care.

6. Drug Discovery and Repurposing:

Bioinformatics and big data analytics have revolutionized the drug discovery process. By analyzing vast datasets containing information on drug-target interactions, chemical structures, and biological pathways, researchers can identify potential drug candidates and predict their efficacy and safety profiles. Computational approaches also enable the repurposing of existing drugs by identifying novel indications based on shared molecular mechanisms. This accelerates the drug development pipeline and enhances therapeutic interventions.

7. Real-world Evidence and Population Health:

Bioinformatics and big data analytics facilitate the analysis of real-world evidence, including data from electronic health records, wearable devices, and population health databases. By harnessing this information, researchers can generate insights into disease prevalence, treatment effectiveness, and healthcare utilization patterns. This knowledge contributes to evidence-based decision-making, public health interventions, and the optimization of healthcare delivery.

8. Collaborative Research and Data Sharing:

Bioinformatics and big data analytics promote collaboration and data sharing among researchers and institutions. By establishing public databases, data repositories, and collaborative platforms, researchers can access and analyze large-scale datasets, fostering interdisciplinary collaborations and accelerating discoveries. This collaborative approach enhances the reproducibility of research findings, maximizes the utilization of available data, and facilitates the translation of research into actionable outcomes.

In summary, bioinformatics and big data analytics play a transformative role in biomedical research. By enabling data integration, genomic analysis, transcriptomics, proteomics, data mining, and the development of predictive models, these fields accelerate discoveries, drive innovation, and improve patient care. As technology continues to advance and datasets expand, the role of bioinformatics and big data analytics will only become more vital in unraveling the complexities of diseases, developing personalized therapies, and transforming healthcare for the benefit of patients worldwide.

Large-Scale Data Analysis and Machine Learning in Biomedical Innovation

In the realm of biomedical innovation, large-scale data analysis and machine learning algorithms have emerged as powerful tools. In this chapter, we will delve into the ways in which these approaches accelerate discoveries and improve patient care, revolutionizing the field of healthcare.

1. Data Integration and Exploration:
Large-scale data analysis allows researchers to integrate diverse datasets from genomics, proteomics, clinical records, and other sources. By combining and exploring these data, researchers can uncover hidden patterns, correlations, and insights that may not be apparent through traditional analysis methods. This integrated approach provides a comprehensive understanding of diseases, identifies novel biomarkers, and reveals potential therapeutic targets.

2. Predictive Modeling and Risk Assessment:
Machine learning algorithms excel at building predictive models from large-scale datasets. By training on vast amounts of patient data, these models can accurately forecast disease progression, treatment responses, and patient outcomes. This information aids

clinicians in making informed decisions regarding treatment strategies and allows for personalized care based on an individual's risk profile.

3. Precision Medicine and Treatment Optimization:

Large-scale data analysis, coupled with machine learning algorithms, supports precision medicine initiatives. By leveraging genomic data, clinical records, and treatment outcomes, researchers can identify molecular signatures associated with specific diseases and treatment responses. This knowledge enables the development of tailored therapies that maximize efficacy while minimizing adverse effects, improving patient outcomes and quality of life.

4. Drug Discovery and Repurposing:

Machine learning algorithms have transformed the drug discovery process. By mining vast amounts of chemical and biological data, these algorithms can identify potential drug candidates and predict their efficacy, toxicity, and side effect profiles. Furthermore, machine learning enables the repurposing of existing drugs by identifying novel indications based on shared molecular mechanisms. This approach expedites the drug development pipeline, reducing costs and time to market.

5. Image Analysis and Diagnostics:

Large-scale data analysis, in conjunction with machine learning, has revolutionized medical imaging and diagnostics. Advanced algorithms can analyze large repositories of medical images, such as MRI scans or histopathology slides, to detect patterns associated with specific diseases. These algorithms can aid in early detection, accurate diagnosis, and prognosis, leading to timely interventions and improved patient outcomes.

6. Real-time Monitoring and Predictive Analytics:

Machine learning algorithms enable real-time monitoring and predictive analytics, particularly in the context of wearable devices and remote patient monitoring. By continuously analyzing data streams from these devices, algorithms can detect anomalies, predict adverse events, and provide timely alerts to healthcare providers. This proactive approach enhances patient safety, reduces hospital admissions, and enables early interventions.

7. Clinical Decision Support Systems:

Machine learning algorithms power clinical decision support systems, which assist healthcare providers in making evidence-based decisions. By integrating patient data, medical literature, and treatment guidelines, these systems can offer personalized recommendations for diagnostics, treatment plans, and medication selection. This support enhances clinical decision-making, reduces errors, and improves patient outcomes.

8. Public Health and Epidemiology:

Large-scale data analysis and machine learning algorithms have a profound impact on public health and epidemiological studies. By analyzing population-level data, such as electronic health records and social media feeds, researchers can identify disease outbreaks, monitor the spread of infectious diseases, and evaluate the effectiveness of public health interventions. These insights enable prompt responses, targeted interventions, and the optimization of public health strategies.

In conclusion, large-scale data analysis and machine learning algorithms have become indispensable tools in biomedical innovation. By enabling data integration, predictive modeling, precision medicine, and drug discovery, these approaches accelerate discoveries and improve patient care. With the continued advancement of technology and the availability of vast datasets, we can expect even greater contributions from large-scale data analysis and machine learning in shaping the future of healthcare and transforming patient outcomes.

Bioinformatics and Big Data in Biomedical Innovation

Bioinformatics, with its application of computational analysis and data management techniques, has made significant contributions to genomics, drug discovery, and clinical decision-making. In this chapter, we will explore examples of how bioinformatics has been applied in these areas, paving the way for transformative advancements in healthcare.

1. Genomics:

a. Genome Assembly and Annotation:
Bioinformatics plays a pivotal role in genome assembly and annotation, the process of deciphering the structure and function of an organism's genome. Through advanced algorithms and computational tools, bioinformaticians can piece together the fragments of DNA sequences generated by high-throughput sequencing technologies. They can then annotate the genes, regulatory elements, and other functional elements within the genome, providing crucial insights into the genetic makeup of organisms and their potential implications in health and disease.

b. Variant Calling and Interpretation:
Bioinformatics enables the identification and interpretation of genetic variants within genomes. By comparing an individual's genomic data to a reference genome, bioinformaticians can pinpoint single nucleotide polymorphisms (SNPs), insertions, deletions, and structural variants. These variants can then be analyzed to determine their potential association with diseases, drug responses, and other phenotypic traits. Bioinformatics tools and databases aid in the interpretation of these variants, providing valuable information for clinical decision-making and personalized medicine.

2. Drug Discovery:

a. Virtual Screening and Molecular Docking:
Bioinformatics facilitates virtual screening and molecular docking, which are computational approaches used in drug discovery. By leveraging large databases of chemical compounds and utilizing molecular modeling techniques, bioinformatics tools can predict the potential binding affinity and interactions between drug candidates and target proteins. This enables researchers to screen and prioritize compounds for further experimental validation, accelerating the drug discovery process and reducing costs.

b. Pharmacogenomics and Drug Response Prediction:
Bioinformatics contributes to pharmacogenomics, the study of how genetic variations influence drug responses. By integrating genomic data with drug response data, bioinformaticians can identify genetic markers associated with variations in drug efficacy, toxicity, and adverse reactions. This information can be used to develop predictive models that aid in personalized medicine, allowing clinicians to select appropriate medications and dosages based on an individual's genetic profile, ultimately improving treatment outcomes and reducing adverse events.

3. Clinical Decision-Making:

a. Clinical Data Integration and Analysis:
Bioinformatics enables the integration and analysis of diverse clinical data, such as electronic health records, imaging data, and patient demographics. By harmonizing and mining these datasets, bioinformaticians can identify patterns, correlations, and associations that help in clinical decision-making. For example, bioinformatics tools can identify clinical features

associated with specific diseases, predict disease progression, or assess treatment responses. This information assists healthcare providers in making evidence-based decisions and tailoring treatment plans to individual patients.

b. Clinical Decision Support Systems:
Bioinformatics plays a crucial role in developing clinical decision support systems (CDSS) that aid healthcare providers in real-time decision-making. By integrating patient data, medical literature, and treatment guidelines, bioinformatics-driven CDSS can provide recommendations for diagnostics, treatment plans, and medication selection, based on individual patient characteristics. These systems enhance clinical decision-making, improve patient safety, and optimize healthcare delivery by providing clinicians with valuable insights and evidence-based guidance.

In summary, bioinformatics has revolutionized genomics, drug discovery, and clinical decision-making by harnessing computational analysis and data management techniques. Through genome assembly and annotation, variant calling and interpretation, virtual screening, pharmacogenomics, and clinical data integration, bioinformatics has accelerated discoveries and improved patient care. As the field continues to advance, bioinformatics will play an increasingly vital role in unraveling the complexities of diseases, discovering new therapeutic targets, and enabling personalized medicine approaches for better healthcare outcomes.

Advancements in Biomedical Devices and Wearable Technologies

In recent years, there have been remarkable advancements in biomedical devices and wearable technologies, transforming the landscape of healthcare. This chapter explores the exciting developments that have revolutionized patient monitoring, diagnostics, treatment delivery, and overall healthcare management.

1. Remote Patient Monitoring:

Biomedical devices and wearables have enabled remote patient monitoring, allowing healthcare providers to monitor patients outside traditional clinical settings. These devices can collect real-time data on vital signs, such as heart rate, blood pressure, and oxygen saturation. This continuous monitoring provides valuable insights into a patient's health status, facilitates early detection of abnormalities, and enables timely interventions. Remote patient monitoring enhances patient care, reduces hospital readmissions, and improves patient outcomes.

2. Continuous Glucose Monitoring (CGM):

CGM systems have transformed the management of diabetes. By utilizing minimally invasive sensors, these wearable devices continuously measure glucose levels in interstitial fluid, eliminating the need for frequent fingerstick tests. CGM systems provide real-time data, allowing individuals with diabetes to monitor their glucose levels closely and make informed decisions about insulin dosing, diet, and physical activity. This technology has improved diabetes management, enhanced glycemic control, and reduced the risk of complications.

3. Smartwatches and Fitness Trackers:

Smartwatches and fitness trackers have gained popularity as wearable devices that monitor various health and fitness parameters. These devices can track steps, distance traveled, calories burned, and sleep patterns. They also incorporate features such as heart rate monitoring, ECG recording, and stress tracking. Smartwatches and fitness trackers empower individuals to monitor their daily activity levels, manage stress, and make informed decisions about their health and well-being.

4. Wearable ECG Monitors:

Wearable electrocardiogram (ECG) monitors have revolutionized cardiac monitoring. These devices, typically worn as patches or wristbands, can record and analyze a person's heart rhythm continuously. Wearable ECG monitors are particularly valuable in detecting arrhythmias, such as atrial fibrillation, which may occur intermittently. They enable early diagnosis, facilitate timely interventions, and improve the management of cardiovascular conditions.

5. Drug Delivery Devices:

Advancements in biomedical devices have led to innovative drug delivery systems. For example, wearable insulin pumps provide continuous subcutaneous insulin infusion for individuals with diabetes, offering precise and personalized insulin delivery. Similarly, wearable patches and transdermal devices enable controlled and targeted drug administration, bypassing the need for frequent injections. These devices improve medication adherence, enhance therapeutic outcomes, and enhance patient convenience.

6. Smart Contact Lenses:

Smart contact lenses represent a cutting-edge development in wearable technology. These lenses integrate sensors to monitor various biomarkers in tears, such as glucose levels for diabetes management or intraocular pressure for glaucoma monitoring. Smart contact lenses provide non-invasive and continuous monitoring, offering valuable data for disease management and early intervention.

7. Assistive Technologies for Disabilities:

Biomedical devices and wearables have expanded assistive technologies for individuals with disabilities. For example, brain-computer interfaces enable communication and control of external devices through neural signals. Prosthetic limbs equipped with sensors and advanced control algorithms allow for more natural and intuitive movements. These technologies improve the quality of life for individuals with disabilities, restoring independence and functionality.

8. Telemedicine and Virtual Care:

The integration of biomedical devices and wearables with telemedicine platforms has revolutionized virtual care delivery. Patients can remotely share data from their wearable devices, enabling healthcare providers to monitor their health status during virtual consultations. This data-driven approach enhances diagnostic accuracy, facilitates remote patient management, and expands access to healthcare services, particularly in underserved areas.

In conclusion, the advancements in biomedical devices and wearable technologies have transformed healthcare by enabling remote patient monitoring, improving disease management, and enhancing overall well-being. From remote patient monitoring and continuous glucose monitoring to smartwatches, wearable

ECG monitors, and smart contact lenses, these technologies have revolutionized patient care, diagnostics, and treatment delivery. As technology continues to advance, we can expect further innovations, leading to more personalized healthcare, improved patient outcomes, and enhanced quality of life.

Role in Remote Patient Monitoring, Early Disease Detection, and Personalized Healthcare Management

Biomedical devices and wearable technologies have played a pivotal role in transforming healthcare by revolutionizing remote patient monitoring, enabling early disease detection, and facilitating personalized healthcare management. In this chapter, we will delve into how these advancements have reshaped these areas of healthcare.

1. Remote Patient Monitoring:

Biomedical devices and wearables have significantly enhanced remote patient monitoring, allowing healthcare providers to monitor patients outside traditional clinical settings. These devices, such as wearable sensors, smartwatches, and connected health devices, can collect real-time data on vital signs, activity levels, sleep patterns, and other relevant health parameters. This continuous monitoring empowers healthcare professionals to track patients' health status remotely, identify potential issues or abnormalities promptly, and intervene in a timely manner. By enabling proactive care and early intervention, remote patient monitoring helps prevent complications, reduces hospital readmissions, and improves patient outcomes.

2. Early Disease Detection:

Biomedical devices and wearables have revolutionized early disease detection by providing continuous monitoring and real-time data analysis. These technologies enable individuals to track and monitor their health parameters, such as heart rate, blood pressure, glucose levels, and other biomarkers, regularly. By analyzing the data collected over time, anomalies and patterns can be identified, potentially indicating the early stages of diseases or health conditions. For example, wearable ECG monitors can detect irregular heart rhythms like atrial fibrillation, allowing for early intervention and management. Early disease detection through biomedical devices and wearables enables timely medical interventions, improves prognosis, and empowers individuals to take proactive steps towards their health.

3. Personalized Healthcare Management:

Biomedical devices and wearables contribute to personalized healthcare management by providing individuals and healthcare providers with valuable data and insights. These devices continuously collect and analyze data related to an individual's health parameters, activity levels, sleep patterns, and more. This wealth of information allows for a deeper understanding of an individual's health profile, enabling personalized interventions, treatment plans, and lifestyle recommendations. For instance, wearable devices can provide personalized exercise recommendations based on an individual's heart rate variability, fitness level, and specific health goals. By tailoring healthcare strategies to individual needs and characteristics, personalized healthcare management can optimize treatment outcomes, improve patient satisfaction, and enhance overall well-being.

4. Data Integration and Decision Support:

Biomedical devices and wearables generate vast amounts of data, and their integration with health information systems and electronic health records is crucial for efficient analysis and decision-making. By integrating wearable-generated data with electronic health records, clinical decision support systems, and artificial intelligence algorithms, healthcare providers can gain a comprehensive view of an individual's health status and make informed decisions. For example, combining wearable data with genomic information can enable personalized medicine approaches, where treatment plans are tailored based on an individual's genetic profile and real-time health data. This integration and data-driven decision support facilitate evidence-based care, enable proactive interventions, and optimize healthcare management.

In summary, biomedical devices and wearable technologies have transformed remote patient monitoring, early disease detection, and personalized healthcare management. Through continuous monitoring, real-time data analysis, and integration with health information systems, these advancements have revolutionized healthcare delivery. By empowering individuals to actively participate in their health management and enabling healthcare providers to monitor patients remotely and make informed decisions, these technologies improve patient outcomes, enhance disease management, and pave the way for a more personalized and proactive approach to healthcare.

Challenges and Future Prospects of Integrating into Mainstream Healthcare

The integration of biomedical devices and wearable technologies into mainstream healthcare brings forth numerous opportunities for improving patient outcomes and transforming healthcare delivery. However, it also presents several challenges that need to be addressed for successful implementation. In this chapter, we will explore these challenges and discuss the future prospects of integrating these technologies into mainstream healthcare.

Challenges:

1. Data Security and Privacy:
With the increasing use of biomedical devices and wearables, the collection and transmission of sensitive health data become paramount. Ensuring robust data security and privacy protection is essential to maintain patient trust and comply with regulatory requirements. Healthcare organizations must implement stringent data protection measures, such as encryption, authentication, and secure data storage, to safeguard patient information from unauthorized access or breaches.

2. Interoperability and Data Standardization:
The integration of diverse biomedical devices and wearables often faces challenges related to interoperability and data standardization. Different devices may use varying data formats, making it difficult to exchange and interpret data seamlessly across different healthcare systems. Establishing standardized protocols and data formats for interoperability is crucial to enable effective data exchange, integration, and analysis,

allowing healthcare providers to make informed decisions based on comprehensive patient information.

3. Integration with Clinical Workflow:

Integrating biomedical devices and wearables into the clinical workflow poses challenges in terms of incorporating these technologies seamlessly into existing healthcare processes. Healthcare providers need to adapt their workflows to accommodate the use of these devices, ensuring that the collected data is effectively utilized in patient care. This may require training healthcare professionals on the use of these technologies, streamlining data integration processes, and integrating the data seamlessly into electronic health records and clinical decision support systems.

4. Validation and Regulation:

As biomedical devices and wearables continue to advance rapidly, it becomes crucial to ensure their safety, efficacy, and accuracy. These technologies need to undergo rigorous validation processes to demonstrate their reliability and precision. Regulatory bodies play a vital role in establishing standards, regulations, and guidelines for these devices to ensure their quality and safety. Continuous monitoring and evaluation of these technologies are necessary to address potential risks and provide reassurance to healthcare providers and patients.

Future Prospects:

1. Enhanced Remote Patient Monitoring:

As technology continues to advance, biomedical devices and wearables will further enhance remote patient monitoring capabilities. Integration with artificial intelligence and machine learning algorithms can enable real-time data analysis, allowing for early detection of health issues and timely interventions. The development of more sophisticated sensors and wearable devices will offer a broader range of health parameters to monitor, providing a comprehensive view of patients' health status.

2. Improved User Experience and Design:

Future advancements in biomedical devices and wearables will focus on improving user experience and design. Smaller, more comfortable, and aesthetically pleasing devices will promote long-term use and adherence. User-friendly interfaces and intuitive applications will simplify data interpretation and encourage active patient engagement in their healthcare management.

3. Precision Medicine and Personalized Care:

The integration of biomedical devices and wearables with genomic information and other biomarkers will drive the development of precision medicine and personalized care. These technologies will enable healthcare providers to tailor treatment plans based on an individual's unique characteristics, genetic profile, and real-time health data. This personalized approach has the potential to optimize treatment outcomes, reduce adverse events, and improve patient satisfaction.

4. Artificial Intelligence and Predictive Analytics:

Artificial intelligence algorithms and predictive analytics will play a significant role in leveraging the vast amount of data generated by biomedical devices and wearables. These technologies can analyze patterns, identify risk factors, and provide predictive insights for disease prevention and management. By harnessing the power of AI, healthcare providers can make data-driven decisions, improve diagnostic accuracy, and enhance patient care.

In conclusion, integrating biomedical devices and wearable technologies into mainstream healthcare presents both challenges and promising future prospects. Overcoming data security concerns, ensuring interoperability, integrating devices into clinical workflows, and addressing regulatory requirements are crucial for successful implementation. Looking ahead, advancements in remote patient monitoring, user experience, precision medicine, and AI-driven analytics hold immense potential to revolutionize healthcare, enhance patient outcomes, and improve the overall quality of care.

Bioprinting and Regenerative Medicine

Emerging Trends and Future Directions in Biomedical Innovation

Bioprinting and regenerative medicine have emerged as transformative fields in biomedical innovation, offering tremendous potential for advancing healthcare and revolutionizing the treatment of various medical conditions. In this chapter, we will explore the emerging trends and future directions in these exciting areas of research and development.

1. Bioink Development and Biomaterials:

One of the key emerging trends in bioprinting is the development of novel bioinks and biomaterials. Bioinks serve as the "ink" in bioprinting processes, providing the structural support and environment necessary for the growth and maturation of cells. Researchers are actively working on developing bioinks that mimic the properties of native tissues, such as their mechanical strength, biocompatibility, and biofunctionality. The incorporation of bioactive molecules, growth factors, and signaling molecules into bioinks is being explored to enhance the regenerative potential of printed constructs. Future advancements in bioink development will lead to more accurate replication of complex tissue structures and improved functional outcomes.

2. Vascularization and Tissue Integration:

Creating vascular networks within printed tissues and organs is a critical challenge in bioprinting. The ability to print intricate and functional blood vessel networks is essential for ensuring proper oxygen and nutrient supply to the cells within the printed constructs. Researchers are exploring various strategies, such as incorporating sacrificial materials or biofabrication techniques that enable the formation of vascular channels. Advancements in vascularization methods will pave the way for the successful printing of larger and more complex tissues and organs with enhanced functionality and integration.

3. Multi-material and Multicellular Printing:

The ability to print structures composed of multiple materials and incorporate diverse cell types is an emerging trend in bioprinting. This approach enables the creation of complex tissue architectures and facilitates the formation of functional interfaces between different cell types. By precisely controlling the placement and composition of different materials and cells within printed constructs, researchers aim to mimic the intricate cellular organization and interactions found in native tissues. Advancements in multi-material and multicellular printing will contribute to the development of more realistic tissue models and the generation of functional tissues and organs for transplantation.

4. Bioprinting of Complex Organs:

While bioprinting has made significant progress in printing simple tissues and organoids, the bioprinting of complex organs remains a major challenge. However, recent research has shown promising results in the bioprinting of more complex structures, such as the heart, liver, and kidney. Techniques like organ-on-a-chip and biofabrication using multiple cell types and support structures are being explored to recreate the complexity and functionality of these organs. The future direction of bioprinting involves advancing these techniques to achieve the successful printing of fully functional, transplantable organs, addressing the critical shortage of donor organs for transplantation.

5. Personalized Medicine and Patient-Specific Constructs:

The concept of personalized medicine is gaining momentum in bioprinting and regenerative medicine. The ability to create patient-specific constructs using a patient's own cells holds immense potential for personalized treatment approaches. Advances in imaging technologies, such as 3D scanning and bioprinting, allow for the creation of patient-specific anatomical models and personalized implants. By tailoring the printed constructs to match the patient's unique anatomy and biology, personalized medicine approaches can improve treatment outcomes, reduce the risk of rejection, and enhance patient satisfaction.

6. Integration of Bioprinting with Other Technologies:

The integration of bioprinting with other cutting-edge technologies is an exciting area of exploration. For example, combining bioprinting with gene editing techniques like CRISPR-Cas9 can enable precise modifications in printed tissues and organs, opening up new avenues for regenerative medicine. Additionally, the integration of bioprinting with microfluidics, nanotechnology, and biofabrication techniques allows for the development of advanced tissue models and disease-on-a-chip platforms for drug discovery and personalized medicine applications.

In conclusion, the field of bioprinting and regenerative medicine is witnessing remarkable progress, and several exciting trends and future directions are shaping the landscape of biomedical innovation. Advancements in bioink development, vascularization, multi-material printing, complex organ bioprinting, personalized medicine, and integration with other technologies hold immense potential for revolutionizing healthcare. As researchers continue to push the boundaries of what is possible, we can anticipate significant breakthroughs in bioprinting and regenerative medicine, leading to improved patient care, enhanced organ transplantation options, and the development of patient-specific therapies.

Potential Applications of 3D Bioprinting

In recent years, 3D bioprinting has emerged as a groundbreaking technology with the potential to revolutionize organ transplantation, tissue regeneration, and drug testing. This chapter explores the exciting applications of 3D bioprinting in these areas of biomedical research and development.

1. Organ Transplantation:

One of the most promising applications of 3D bioprinting is in the field of organ transplantation. The shortage of donor organs for transplantation is a critical issue worldwide, leading to long waiting lists and a significant number of patient deaths. 3D bioprinting offers a potential solution by enabling the fabrication of patient-specific organs or tissues using a patient's own cells. By precisely depositing layers of bioink containing different cell types, bioprinters can create complex organ structures with the potential to function and integrate with the patient's body. This approach has the potential to overcome issues of organ rejection and the need for immunosuppressive drugs, significantly improving the success rates of organ transplantation.

2. Tissue Regeneration:

3D bioprinting holds great promise for tissue regeneration by providing a means to create complex, three-dimensional structures that mimic the architecture and functionality of native tissues. By printing layers of bioink containing various cell types, growth factors, and biomaterials, researchers can create tissue constructs that promote cell growth, differentiation, and tissue integration. This technology has the potential to regenerate damaged or diseased tissues, such as cartilage, bone, skin, and even more complex structures like blood vessels and heart tissue. Bioprinted tissues can be used for transplantation, reconstructive surgery, or as models for studying disease progression and drug discovery.

3. Drug Testing and Development:

Another significant application of 3D bioprinting is in the field of drug testing and development. Traditional two-dimensional cell culture models often fail to accurately represent the complexity of human tissues and organs, leading to limited predictive capabilities for drug efficacy and toxicity. Bioprinting allows for the creation of more realistic three-dimensional tissue models that closely resemble the native tissue microenvironment. These models can be used to test the safety and effectiveness of drugs, identify potential toxicities, and understand the underlying mechanisms of drug action. Bioprinted tissues can also be used to develop personalized medicine approaches, where drug responses can be tested on patient-specific tissue constructs, improving treatment outcomes and reducing adverse effects.

4. Disease Modeling:

3D bioprinting enables the creation of disease models that closely mimic the characteristics of specific diseases, providing valuable tools for studying disease progression and developing targeted therapies. By incorporating patient-specific cells and disease-specific biomarkers into bioprinted tissue constructs, researchers can recreate the complex cellular interactions and microenvironment that contribute to disease development. These models can be used to study disease mechanisms, test potential therapies, and identify novel drug targets. Disease-on-a-chip platforms, created by integrating bioprinted tissues with microfluidics, allow for the simulation of physiological conditions and dynamic cellular responses, further enhancing the accuracy of disease models.

5. Surgical Planning and Training:

Bioprinting can also be utilized for surgical planning and training purposes. By using patient-specific imaging data, bioprinters can create anatomically accurate models of organs or tissues, helping surgeons visualize and plan complex surgical procedures. These models can aid in optimizing surgical approaches, reducing operating time, and improving patient outcomes. Additionally, bioprinted tissue models can be used for surgical training, allowing surgeons to practice procedures on realistic, patient-specific replicas.

In conclusion, 3D bioprinting has the potential to transform organ transplantation, tissue regeneration, and drug testing. The ability to create patient-specific organs and tissues, replicate complex tissue architectures, and mimic disease conditions opens up new avenues for personalized medicine, improved treatment outcomes, and more accurate drug testing. As the technology continues to advance, we can expect exciting developments in the field of 3D bioprinting, leading to enhanced patient care, reduced healthcare burdens, and significant advancements in regenerative medicine and pharmaceutical research.

Bioprinting and Regenerative Medicine

Ethical Considerations and Future Directions of Bioprinting Technology

As bioprinting technology continues to advance, it brings with it a range of ethical considerations that must be carefully addressed. In this chapter, we will highlight some of these ethical considerations and explore the future directions of bioprinting technology.

1. Ethical Considerations in Bioprinting:

a. Source of Cells and Tissues: Bioprinting requires a source of cells and tissues to create constructs. The ethical considerations arise when considering the source of these materials. The use of human cells raises questions about informed consent, privacy, and the potential exploitation of vulnerable populations. Additionally, the use of animal cells or tissues may raise concerns about animal welfare and the ethical implications of using animals in research.

b. Intellectual Property: Bioprinting involves the use of advanced technologies and techniques that may be subject to intellectual property rights. Ethical questions arise regarding the accessibility and affordability of bioprinting technologies, as well as the equitable distribution of benefits derived from bioprinted products.

c. Safety and Regulation: As bioprinting moves towards clinical applications, ensuring the safety, efficacy, and regulatory compliance of bioprinted products becomes paramount. Ethical considerations include the need for rigorous testing, transparent reporting of results, and adherence to established regulatory frameworks to minimize risks to patients and ensure the ethical conduct of research.

d. Equity and Access: Bioprinting has the potential to revolutionize healthcare, but ethical concerns arise regarding equitable access to bioprinted products and therapies. Ensuring that the benefits of bioprinting are accessible to all individuals, regardless of socioeconomic status or geographic location, is crucial to avoid exacerbating existing health disparities.

2. Future Directions in Bioprinting:

a. Complex Organ Printing: Bioprinting is advancing towards the goal of printing complex organs with intricate vascular networks. Future directions involve refining the techniques and materials used to create functional vascular networks within printed organs. This would overcome one of the major challenges in organ transplantation and significantly improve the success rates of printed organs.

b. Bioink Development: The development of advanced bioinks with tailored properties is an area of ongoing research. Future directions involve exploring novel biomaterials, optimizing the composition of bioinks, and incorporating bioactive molecules to enhance the regenerative potential of printed constructs. This would enable the creation of more realistic and functional tissues for transplantation and regenerative medicine applications.

c. Personalized Medicine: Bioprinting holds great promise for personalized medicine. Future directions involve using patient-specific cells and imaging data to create customized tissue constructs for transplantation, disease modeling, and drug testing. This approach has the potential to improve treatment outcomes, reduce adverse effects, and advance precision medicine approaches.

d. Ethical Frameworks and Governance: As bioprinting technology advances, the development of robust ethical frameworks and governance structures becomes crucial. Future directions involve establishing guidelines and regulations to address the ethical considerations associated with bioprinting, ensuring responsible research and development, equitable access, and the protection of individuals' rights and welfare.

e. Collaboration and Interdisciplinary Research: Bioprinting is a highly interdisciplinary field. Future directions involve fostering collaboration between scientists, engineers, ethicists, policymakers, and other stakeholders to collectively address the ethical challenges and guide the responsible development and implementation of bioprinting technology.

In conclusion, bioprinting technology holds immense potential in regenerative medicine. However, it is essential to proactively address the ethical considerations associated with this technology. By ensuring transparency, open dialogue, and the development of robust ethical frameworks, we can navigate these challenges and shape the future directions of bioprinting in a responsible and equitable manner.
s.

Future Directions and Challenges in Biomedical Innovation

Emerging Trends and Future Directions in Biomedical Innovation

Biomedical innovation continues to advance at a rapid pace, opening up new possibilities for improving healthcare outcomes and addressing global health challenges. In this chapter, we will discuss some of the emerging trends and future directions in biomedical innovation.

1. Precision Medicine:

Precision medicine is an emerging field that aims to tailor medical treatments and interventions to individual patients based on their unique genetic makeup, lifestyle, and environment. Advances in genomics, proteomics, and other 'omics' technologies have provided valuable insights into the underlying molecular mechanisms of diseases, enabling more targeted and personalized approaches to diagnosis, treatment, and prevention. The future of precision medicine lies in the integration of multi-omics data, advanced computational algorithms, and artificial intelligence (AI) to develop predictive models and personalized treatment plans. This approach has the potential to revolutionize healthcare by improving treatment efficacy, reducing adverse effects, and optimizing patient outcomes.

2. Artificial Intelligence and Machine Learning:

Artificial intelligence (AI) and machine learning (ML) are playing an increasingly significant role in biomedical innovation. AI algorithms can analyze vast amounts of healthcare data, including electronic health records, medical images, and genomics data, to identify patterns, make predictions, and support clinical decision-making. ML algorithms can assist in disease diagnosis, drug discovery, and treatment optimization. The future of AI and ML in biomedical innovation involves the development of more sophisticated algorithms, the integration of diverse datasets, and the establishment of robust ethical frameworks to ensure the responsible and ethical use of AI in healthcare.

3. Digital Health and Wearable Devices:

Digital health technologies and wearable devices have gained significant attention in recent years. These technologies, such as fitness trackers, smartwatches, and mobile health applications, enable the collection of real-time health data and facilitate remote monitoring and management of patients' health conditions. The future direction of digital health lies in the integration of these technologies with AI, ML, and Internet of Things (IoT) to create a seamless and interconnected healthcare ecosystem. This includes the development of advanced sensors, improved data privacy and security measures, and the utilization of data analytics to derive meaningful insights for personalized healthcare interventions.

4. Nanomedicine and Drug Delivery Systems:

Nanomedicine involves the use of nanotechnology for medical diagnosis, imaging, and targeted drug delivery. Nanoparticles and nanocarriers can be designed to deliver drugs specifically to diseased tissues, reducing systemic side effects and improving therapeutic efficacy. The future of nanomedicine lies in the development of innovative nanomaterials, smart drug delivery systems, and nanosensors for early disease detection and monitoring. Additionally, the integration of nanotechnology with other emerging fields, such as regenerative medicine and gene editing, holds great promise for the development of novel therapeutic strategies.

5. Global Health and Access to Healthcare:

Addressing global health challenges and improving access to healthcare is a crucial future direction in biomedical innovation. This involves developing affordable and scalable solutions, especially for low-resource settings. Innovations in point-of-care diagnostics, telemedicine, and low-cost medical devices can help bridge healthcare disparities and ensure equitable access to quality healthcare worldwide. Collaboration between researchers, policymakers, and healthcare providers is essential to identify and address the unique challenges faced by different regions and populations.

6. Ethical Considerations and Regulatory Frameworks:

As biomedical innovation progresses, it is crucial to address the ethical, legal, and social implications associated with emerging technologies. Future directions involve the development of robust ethical frameworks and regulatory guidelines to ensure the responsible and ethical use of innovative technologies. This includes issues related to privacy, data security, consent, equity, and transparency. Stakeholder engagement and public dialogue are vital to navigate these challenges and develop inclusive and socially responsible biomedical innovations.

In conclusion, biomedical innovation is evolving rapidly, driven by advances in technology, data analytics, and interdisciplinary collaboration. The emerging trends and future directions discussed in this chapter hold great promise for transforming healthcare delivery, improving patient outcomes, and addressing global health challenges. By embracing these trends and addressing associated challenges, we can shape a future where healthcare is more personalized, accessible, and effective.

Challenges and Barriers in Translating Research into Clinical Practice

While biomedical research holds great promise for advancing healthcare, translating research findings into clinical practice poses several challenges and barriers. In this chapter, we will explore some of these challenges and discuss the barriers that researchers and healthcare practitioners face in translating research into clinical applications.

1. Time and Cost:

Translating research findings into clinical practice is a time-consuming and costly process. It typically involves several stages, including preclinical studies, clinical trials, regulatory approval, and market adoption. Each stage requires significant financial resources, infrastructure, and dedicated personnel. The lengthy timelines and high costs associated with translating research can impede the progress and implementation of innovative technologies and therapies.

2. Complex Regulatory Environment:

The regulatory environment surrounding the approval and commercialization of new medical interventions is complex and stringent. Researchers and companies must navigate through a maze of regulatory requirements, including safety and efficacy assessments, ethical considerations, and compliance with Good Clinical Practice (GCP) guidelines. Meeting these regulatory standards can be challenging and time-consuming, often requiring extensive documentation, rigorous testing, and close collaboration with regulatory authorities.

3. Limited Generalizability:

Research studies often focus on specific populations or controlled settings, which may limit the generalizability of the findings to broader clinical practice. Factors such as patient diversity, comorbidities, and variations in healthcare settings can impact the effectiveness and applicability of research outcomes in real-world scenarios. Bridging the gap between research and clinical practice requires conducting studies that reflect the diversity of patient populations and considering real-world complexities to ensure the successful translation of research findings.

4. Resistance to Change:

The healthcare system is complex and conservative, and adopting new research findings and technologies can face resistance from various stakeholders. Healthcare providers may be hesitant to adopt new interventions due to concerns about efficacy, safety, cost, or changes in established practices. Additionally, patients and the public may have limited awareness or skepticism about novel treatments or may prefer traditional approaches. Overcoming resistance to change requires robust evidence, effective communication, and stakeholder engagement to build trust and encourage the adoption of innovative practices.

5. Interdisciplinary Collaboration:

Translating research into clinical practice often requires interdisciplinary collaboration among researchers, clinicians, industry partners, and policymakers. However, fostering effective collaboration across different disciplines and sectors can be challenging. Differences in language, priorities, and incentives can hinder effective communication and collaboration.

Encouraging and supporting interdisciplinary teamwork, establishing platforms for knowledge exchange, and promoting a shared vision of patient-centered care are crucial for successful translation of research findings.

6. Funding and Investment:

Securing funding for translational research and development can be a significant barrier. Traditional funding mechanisms may prioritize basic research over translational efforts, making it challenging for researchers to access the necessary resources to move their findings from the lab to clinical practice. Additionally, attracting investment from the private sector may be challenging if the market potential or return on investment is uncertain. Addressing funding gaps and establishing funding mechanisms that incentivize translational research can help overcome this barrier.

7. Data Integration and Interoperability:

Translating research findings into clinical practice often requires the integration and analysis of diverse datasets, including electronic health records, genomics data, and imaging data. However, data interoperability and integration remain significant challenges in healthcare systems. Fragmented data systems, privacy concerns, and technical barriers can impede the seamless flow of information and hinder the translation of research findings into actionable insights. Developing robust health information exchange systems and promoting data sharing standards are critical for effective translation of research into clinical practice.

In conclusion, translating research findings into clinical practice is a complex and multifaceted process. Overcoming the challenges and barriers discussed in this chapter requires collaborative efforts between researchers, clinicians, policymakers, and industry partners. By addressing issues related to funding, regulation, data integration, and stakeholder engagement, we can accelerate the translation of innovative research into clinical applications, ultimately improving patient care and outcomes.

The Importance of Collaboration between Academia, Industry, and Regulatory Bodies for Continued Progress

Collaboration between academia, industry, and regulatory bodies plays a crucial role in driving continued progress in biomedical innovation. In this chapter, we will highlight the importance of collaboration among these stakeholders and discuss how their collective efforts can foster innovation, accelerate development, and ensure the safe and effective translation of scientific discoveries into tangible healthcare solutions.

1. Knowledge Exchange:

Academic institutions are at the forefront of scientific research, generating new knowledge and insights into diseases, therapeutic approaches, and innovative technologies. Collaboration with industry allows for the transfer of academic research into the development of practical applications. Industry partners bring expertise in product development, manufacturing, and commercialization, translating academic discoveries into tangible products and technologies that can benefit patients. By sharing knowledge and expertise, academia and industry can bridge the gap between fundamental research and real-world applications.

2. Translational Research:

Translational research aims to bridge the gap between basic scientific discoveries and clinical applications. Collaboration between academia, industry, and regulatory bodies is essential for successful translational research. Academic researchers contribute their scientific expertise and experimental findings, while industry partners provide resources, infrastructure, and practical insights into product development and commercialization. Regulatory bodies play a critical role in ensuring that translational research adheres to safety and efficacy standards. By working together, these stakeholders can streamline the translation of research findings into clinical practice, bringing new therapies and technologies to patients faster.

3. Innovation and Commercialization:

Collaboration between academia and industry fosters a culture of innovation and entrepreneurship. Academic researchers often possess deep scientific knowledge and expertise, while industry partners bring business acumen and resources to navigate the complex commercialization process. By collaborating, these stakeholders can identify promising research discoveries with commercial potential, secure funding for development, and navigate regulatory pathways for market approval. This collaboration not only accelerates the commercialization of innovations but also facilitates the development of sustainable business models that can support future research and development efforts.

4. Regulatory Compliance and Patient Safety:

Regulatory bodies play a vital role in ensuring the safety and efficacy of medical interventions. Collaboration between academia, industry, and regulatory bodies is essential for navigating the complex regulatory landscape. Academic researchers and industry partners can work together to generate robust scientific evidence and data required for regulatory approval. Regulatory bodies, on the other hand, provide guidance, oversight, and expertise in evaluating the safety and efficacy of new therapies and technologies. By collaborating closely, these stakeholders can ensure that innovative biomedical products meet rigorous standards and prioritize patient safety.

5. Policy Development and Advocacy:

Collaboration between academia, industry, and regulatory bodies also extends to policy development and advocacy. These stakeholders can work together to shape policies that promote innovation, support research funding, and create a favorable environment for the development and adoption of new therapies and technologies. By advocating for policies that encourage collaboration, remove barriers, and provide incentives for innovation, academia, industry, and regulatory bodies can collectively drive progress and improve healthcare outcomes.

6. Continuous Learning and Improvement:

Collaboration among academia, industry, and regulatory bodies facilitates continuous learning and improvement. Academic researchers can learn from industry partners about the practical challenges and considerations involved in translating research into clinical applications. Industry partners can gain insights from academia about the latest scientific advancements and emerging research areas. Regulatory bodies can learn from both academia and industry to adapt regulatory frameworks and guidelines to keep pace with technological advancements. This collaborative learning environment enables stakeholders to adapt, innovate, and improve strategies for biomedical innovation.

In conclusion, collaboration between academia, industry, and regulatory bodies is vital for driving continued progress in biomedical innovation. By leveraging each stakeholder's unique expertise, resources, and perspectives, these collaborations can accelerate the translation of research findings into clinical practice, promote innovation, ensure regulatory compliance, and ultimately improve patient care and outcomes. Fostering a collaborative ecosystem that encourages knowledge exchange, translational research, innovation, and policy advocacy is crucial for the future of biomedical innovation.

Conclusion

Throughout this book, we have explored various aspects of biomedical innovation, discussing key findings and advancements that have shaped the field. Here, we summarize the key takeaways from our exploration, highlighting the significant progress and promising directions in biomedical research and its impact on healthcare.

1. Advances in Precision Medicine:
Precision medicine has emerged as a transformative approach in healthcare, leveraging advancements in genomics, proteomics, and other omics technologies. These advancements have enabled personalized diagnosis, treatment, and prevention strategies tailored to individual patients, considering their unique genetic makeup, lifestyle, and environmental factors.

2. Breakthroughs in Therapeutic Development:
The development of novel therapies has witnessed remarkable advancements. From targeted therapies and immunotherapies to gene and cell-based therapies, researchers have made significant progress in combating various diseases, including cancer, genetic disorders, and autoimmune conditions. These innovative treatments offer new hope to patients by improving efficacy and reducing side effects.

3. Digital Health and Wearable Technologies:

The integration of digital health technologies, such as wearable devices, remote monitoring systems, and telehealth platforms, has revolutionized healthcare delivery. These technologies enable continuous monitoring, real-time data collection, and remote patient-doctor interactions, enhancing patient engagement, disease management, and preventive care.

4. Artificial Intelligence and Machine Learning:

Artificial intelligence (AI) and machine learning (ML) have become powerful tools in biomedical research and clinical practice. AI algorithms can analyze vast amounts of data, identify patterns, and generate insights that aid in disease diagnosis, drug discovery, and treatment optimization. ML models can improve risk prediction, patient stratification, and personalized treatment recommendations.

5. Advancements in Biomedical Imaging:

Imaging technologies have undergone significant advancements, enabling early and accurate diagnosis of diseases. From high-resolution MRI and PET scans to molecular imaging techniques, researchers have developed non-invasive imaging modalities that provide detailed anatomical and functional information, facilitating precise disease characterization and treatment planning.

6. The Role of Big Data and Data Analytics:

The availability of large-scale, diverse datasets has transformed biomedical research. Big data analytics and bioinformatics tools have enabled researchers to uncover intricate relationships, identify biomarkers, and gain deeper insights into disease mechanisms. This knowledge has the potential to guide personalized treatment decisions and improve patient outcomes.

7. Ethical and Regulatory Considerations:

The rapid pace of biomedical innovation has raised various ethical and regulatory considerations. As we navigate the ethical challenges associated with genetic manipulation, data privacy, and AI-driven decision-making, it becomes crucial to strike a balance between innovation, patient autonomy, and societal well-being. Robust regulatory frameworks and ethical guidelines are essential to ensure the responsible development and deployment of biomedical technologies.

8. Collaborative Ecosystem:

The success of biomedical innovation relies on a collaborative ecosystem that brings together academia, industry, healthcare providers, and regulatory bodies. Collaboration fosters knowledge exchange, accelerates translational research, promotes innovation, and ensures regulatory compliance. By working together, stakeholders can overcome challenges, leverage their unique expertise, and drive continued progress in biomedical research and healthcare.

As we move forward, it is imperative to address the challenges and barriers discussed in this book, such as funding gaps, regulatory complexities, and data interoperability. By doing so, we can unlock the full potential of biomedical innovation and strive towards a future where advanced diagnostics, targeted therapies, and personalized medicine become the standard of care, ultimately improving health outcomes and quality of life for individuals worldwide.

Biomedical innovation holds immense transformative potential in revolutionizing healthcare as we know it. Throughout this book, we have explored the remarkable advancements and breakthroughs in biomedical research, highlighting the profound impact they have on improving patient care and outcomes. In this conclusion, we emphasize the transformative potential of biomedical innovation and its ability to reshape the landscape of healthcare for the better.

1. Personalized Medicine:
Biomedical innovation has paved the way for personalized medicine, shifting healthcare from a one-size-fits-all approach to a tailored, patient-centric model. By leveraging advancements in genomics,

proteomics, and other omics technologies, healthcare providers can now analyze an individual's unique genetic makeup, lifestyle, and environmental factors to deliver precise diagnoses, treatments, and preventive strategies. This personalized approach has the potential to maximize treatment efficacy, minimize adverse effects, and optimize patient outcomes.

2. Targeted Therapies:

The development of targeted therapies has revolutionized the treatment of various diseases, particularly cancer. By identifying specific molecular targets involved in disease progression, researchers have been able to design therapies that selectively attack diseased cells while sparing healthy tissues. This targeted approach improves treatment efficacy and reduces the toxic side effects associated with traditional treatments, leading to better patient tolerability and quality of life.

3. Innovative Treatment Modalities:

Biomedical innovation has introduced a plethora of innovative treatment modalities that were once considered science fiction. From gene and cell-based therapies to immunotherapies and regenerative medicine, researchers have made significant strides in developing novel approaches to tackle previously untreatable or incurable conditions. These groundbreaking therapies offer new hope to patients, potentially transforming devastating diseases into manageable chronic conditions or even providing complete cures.

4. Digital Health Technologies:

The integration of digital health technologies has brought about a paradigm shift in healthcare delivery. Wearable devices, remote monitoring systems, and telehealth platforms enable continuous and real-time monitoring of patients, facilitating early detection of health issues and timely interventions. These technologies empower individuals to take an active role in managing their health, promote preventive care, and enable remote access to healthcare services, particularly for underserved populations. The democratization of healthcare through digital technologies has the potential to improve access, reduce healthcare costs, and enhance overall population health.

5. Data-Driven Insights:

The abundance of data and advancements in data analytics have unlocked a wealth of insights into disease mechanisms, treatment responses, and population health trends. By leveraging big data analytics, artificial intelligence, and machine learning, researchers can identify patterns, discover novel biomarkers, and develop predictive models for disease diagnosis, prognosis, and treatment optimization.

These data-driven insights have the potential to revolutionize clinical decision-making, enabling healthcare providers to deliver more precise, evidence-based care tailored to individual patients.

6. Revolutionizing Medical Imaging:

Advancements in biomedical imaging technologies have transformed the way we visualize and diagnose diseases. High-resolution imaging modalities, such as MRI, CT, and molecular imaging techniques, provide detailed anatomical and functional information, enabling accurate and early detection of diseases. This early diagnosis facilitates timely interventions, improves treatment outcomes, and reduces healthcare costs. Additionally, imaging technologies play a crucial role in guiding minimally invasive procedures, improving surgical accuracy, and monitoring treatment responses.

7. Enhanced Collaboration and Interdisciplinary Approaches:

Biomedical innovation thrives through collaboration and interdisciplinary approaches. The convergence of diverse fields, including biology, engineering, computer science, and data analytics, enables researchers to tackle complex healthcare challenges from multiple angles. Collaborative efforts between academia, industry, healthcare providers, and regulatory bodies foster knowledge exchange, accelerate research translation, and promote the development and adoption of innovative solutions.

In conclusion, biomedical innovation has the transformative potential to revolutionize healthcare by advancing personalized medicine, introducing targeted therapies, embracing digital health technologies, harnessing data-driven insights, revolutionizing medical imaging, and promoting collaboration among diverse stakeholders. By embracing and supporting these advancements, we can usher in an era of healthcare that is more precise, effective, accessible, and patient-centered. The future holds immense promise as we continue to push the boundaries of biomedical innovation, ultimately improving health outcomes and positively impacting the lives of individuals worldwide.

About the Author

Dr. Maya Thompson is a renowned expert in the field of biomedical innovation. With a passion for advancing healthcare solutions, Dr. Thompson has dedicated her career to pushing the boundaries of medical research and technology.

Dr. Thompson holds a Ph.D. in Biomedical Engineering from a prestigious institution and has extensive experience collaborating with interdisciplinary teams to develop groundbreaking solutions. Her research contributions have led to significant advancements in areas such as medical devices, regenerative medicine, and diagnostic tools.

As a respected thought leader, Dr. Thompson has been invited to speak at international conferences and has published numerous scholarly articles in reputable scientific journals. She is known for her ability to communicate complex scientific concepts in a clear and accessible manner, making her work relatable to both experts and enthusiasts in the field.

Driven by a desire to bridge the gap between academia and industry, Dr. Thompson actively engages with startups, healthcare organizations, and government institutions to promote the translation of innovative ideas into practical applications. Through her consulting work, she helps guide entrepreneurs and researchers in navigating the intricacies of biomedical innovation, supporting them in bringing life-changing solutions to market.

In "Biomedical Innovation," Dr. Maya Thompson shares her wealth of knowledge and experience, guiding readers through the dynamic landscape of biomedical research and development. With a focus on fostering creativity, collaboration, and ethical practices, Dr. Thompson empowers readers to explore the forefront of biomedical innovation and make a positive impact on the future of healthcare.

Through her writing, Dr. Thompson aims to inspire the next generation of biomedical pioneers, encouraging them to embrace curiosity, think critically, and leverage cutting-edge technologies to drive transformative change in the field.